The Ketogenic diet for beginners: 25 best quick and easy recipes for weight loss.

Mia Kendal

© **Copyright 2016 – Mia Kendal - All rights reserved.**

In no way is it legal to reproduce, duplicate, or transmit any part of this document in either electronic means or in printed format. Recording of this publication is strictly prohibited and any storage of this document is not allowed unless with written permission from the publisher. All rights reserved.

The information provided herein is stated to be truthful and consistent, in that any liability, in terms of inattention or otherwise, by any usage or abuse of any policies, processes, or directions contained within is the solitary and utter responsibility of the recipient reader. Under no circumstances will any legal responsibility or blame be held against the publisher for any reparation, damages, or monetary loss due to the information herein, either directly or indirectly.

Legal Notice:

This book is copyright protected. This is only for personal use. You cannot amend, distribute, sell, use, quote or paraphrase any part or the content within this book without the consent of the author or copyright owner. Legal action will be pursued if this is breached.

Disclaimer Notice:

Please note the information contained within this document is for educational and entertainment purposes only. Every attempt has been made to provide accurate, up to date and reliable complete information. No warranties of any kind are expressed or implied. Readers acknowledge that the author is not engaging in the rendering of legal, financial, medical or professional advice.

By reading this document, the reader agrees that under no circumstances are we responsible for any losses, direct or indirect, which are incurred as a result of the use of information contained within this document, including, but not limited to, —errors, omissions, or inaccuracies.

Contents

Introduction 1

Chapter 1: Introducing You To The World Of The Ketogenic Diet 2

    The definition of Ketogenic Diet 2

    Know your Keto ingredients 3

    Health Benefits Of A Ketogenic Diet 4

    The physical effects on the body 5

    Some negative effects of a Keto diet 6

Chapter 2: Start Your Day With These Keto Breakfast Meals 7

    Keto Breakfast Tacos 7

    Breakfast Keto Pizza Waffles 9

    Keto Breakfast Burger 10

    Mini Pancake Donuts 12

    Cinnamon Roll Oatmeal 13

    Ham And Cheddar Chive Soufflé 15

    Blackberry Pudding 17

Chapter 3: The Delightful Luncheon Recipes For Keto Lovers 19

    Bacon Avocado And Chicken Sandwich 19

    Cheese Stuffed Bacon Wrapped Hot Dogs 21

Crispy Tofu and Bok Choy Salad 22

Nasi Lemak 24

Jalapeno Popper Mug Cake 26

Chicken Enchilada Soup 28

Thai Peanut Shrimp Curry 29

Chapter 4: Meals For When You Are About To Sleep, Your Dinner 32

Keto Sushi 32

Walnut Crusted Salmon 33

Slow Cooker Braised Oxtail 35

Nacho Chicken Casserole 36

Ketogenic Grilled Short Ribs 38

Oven Baked Turkey Leg 40

Italian Stuffed Meatballs 42

Chapter 5: A Few Desserts For The Sweet Tooth Out There 44

Mini Vanilla Cloud Cupcakes 44

Bake Free Coconut Cashew Bars 46

Choco Peanut Tarts 47

Pumpkin Pecan Pie Ice Cream 49

Conclusion 51

Introduction

I am highly honored that you have deiced to download this book and support me in spreading the word of the Ketogenic diet and help people all across the world to know about the wonderful benefits of a Ketogenic diet.

This book does not only aim to act as a recipe book, but also as an initial kick starting guideline for those who are absolutely unfamiliar with this topic.

Throughout the eBook, you will be introduced to the very concepts of the Ketogenic diet and understand why the whole world is suddenly altering their way of life into following a more Ketogenic standard. With this, you will be given step by step methods on creating some of the more delicious and easy to make Keto recipes out there to start off your journey.

The only thing you will need to remember before embarking on your quest is that if you decide to ultimately follow the path to becoming a Ketogenic follower, you are going to need to be consistent all the way through.

A simple heavy snack once in a while doesn't matter, but don't turn that into a habit and deviate too much from your proper course.

I congratulate you on being daring enough to take on this life changing step and I wholeheartedly wish that may you be able to acquire all of the health benefits which a Ketogenic diet has to offer!

Chapter 1: Introducing You To The World Of The Ketogenic Diet

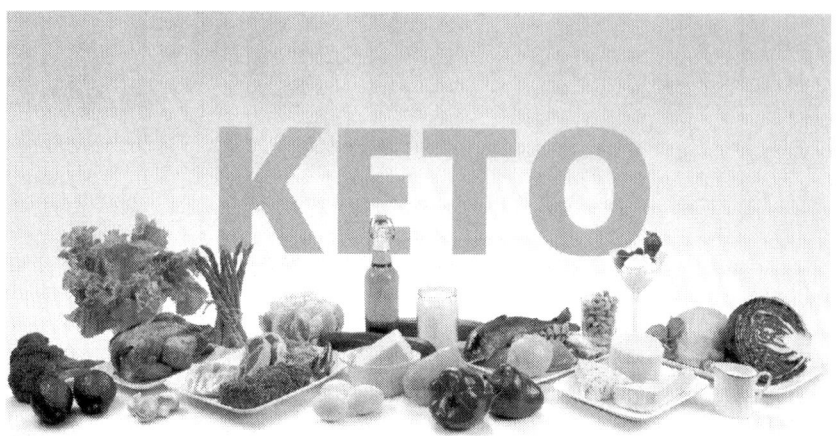

You have most definitely heard of the term "Ketogenic" whenever the topic of healthy diet pops up! If you an amateur in this field, the term might induce a sense of sudden confusion inside you.

Let's start our book from the very basics and explain what the term actually means.

The definition of Ketogenic Diet

The key word here to notice is "Keto" which is primarily derived from the human body's metabolic process known as Ketosis, which produces Ketones.

A Keto diet is essentially a strict diet plan which aims to lower the carbohydrate intake of the body. It has been synonymously known as a low carb high fat diet, low carb diet, etc. For our book, we are simply going to be referring to it as a Ketogenic diet.

Whenever our body is exposed to something that is high

in carbohydrate contents, the production of glucose and insulin in our body tends to increase.

Now, you should understand here that glucose is the most easily convertible molecule in our body so, given the chance, the body will always try to use glucose to acquire the energy required for day to day activities.

Insulin on the other hand can be thought of as being a companion molecule in our blood stream which helps to process the glucose in our body. Since the body tends to use glucose as its core energy source, the fats in our body are not necessarily required to be broken down and so are often stored around the body.

When you are going through a higher carbohydrate diet, the body will therefore burn less fat and keep using glucose as its energy source.

When the consumption of carbohydrates is lowered, the body tends to alter its internal conditions and go to a phase called "ketosis". This is nothing to be alarmed of! It's just simply the body's natural response to deal with a lower food intake. During this state, the body is forced to produce a greater number of ketones which helps the body to break down fat.

So, if observed closely, the ultimate goal of going through a low carb Ketogenic diet plan is essentially to influence the body into ketosis so that our body starts to burn fat instead of glucose.

Know your Keto ingredients

To start off a Ketogenic diet, it is highly essential that you create an outline inside your head. The dishes which you are typically required to eat during your diet will largely depend on the strictness of your diet plan. You are going to need to bring factors such as "How fast do you want to burn your fat?" or "How fast do you want your body to attain ketosis?" into account. Generally speaking, the recommended levels for a strict Keto diet requires less than <15g of carbs per day. On the other hand, you can also go for 20-30g carbs normally.

Below is a list of some of the common vegetables and their carb content which you might be interested in.

Vegetable	Amount	Net Carbs
Spinach (Raw)	1/2 Cup	0.1
Bok Choi	1/2 Cup	0.2
Lettuce (Romaine)	1/2 Cup	0.2
Broccoli (Florets)	1/2 Cup	0.8
Cauliflower (Steamed)	1/2 Cup	0.9
Cabbage (Green Raw)	1/2 Cup	1.1
Cauliflower (Raw)	1/2 Cup	1.4
Collard Greens	1/2 Cup	2
Kale steamed	1/2 Cup	2.1
Green Beans steamed	1/2 Cup	2.9

Health Benefits Of A Ketogenic Diet

The list of health benefits which a human can enjoy if a proper Ketogenic diet is followed is almost limitless. But here are some of the more prominent ones which you should know about during your early stages:

- A nice Ketogenic diet is proven to lower the levels of cholesterol by encouraging the buildup of triglycerides which helps to reduce arterial blockages.
- Since the body will be using the stored fat as its primary source of energy while in ketosis, weight loss will be highly encouraged.
- The decrease of LDL during the state of ketosis will help in reducing the blood sugar levels, directly mitigating the chances of suffering from type 2 diabetes.
- Since fat is pretty much all over our body, it will act as a much more efficient and reliable source of energy for our body. This in turn will help you to feel much more energetic and pumped up throughout the day.
- The feeling of hunger will be lessened.
- Recently it has been proved that ketosis apparently also decreases the levels of skin inflammation and production of acne lesions in the skin.

The physical effects on the body

Going in for a completely different style of diet, as with anything else, will take some time for the body to habituate itself to. After the first few weeks of your diet, once the body senses that it is going to be exposed to a certain type of food each and every day, it will be able to prepare itself beforehand by building up a set of enzymes specifically readied for the purpose of processing Keto meals and inducing ketosis.

It should be noted though that during the early stages of a Keto diet, you might experience some of the following symptoms, including a general sense of lethargy. Don't be alarmed as these are pretty normal. Once the body gets used to it, they will eventually go away.

- Mental fogginess
- Headaches
- Keto flu
- Aggravation
- Dizziness

Ketosis encourages the body to flush out a large amount of electrolytes from the body which causes these effects in the first place. To tackle the diuretic effect, it is suggested that you increase your water consumption during a Keto diet. Another unusual piece of advice would be to increase your salt input as well which will help to replenish the electrolytes.

The adaptation process usually take 1 week at least and 2 weeks at best if done properly.

Some negative effects of a Keto diet

Everything these days is a two sided coin. The Ketogenic diet doesn't escape from that trend either. While in general the positive effects of the Ketogenic diet is tenfold, there are still some factors which you should be aware of, including:
- If you ever decide to quit the Keto diet while having stuck with the routine for a long time previously, you might face some weight gain and health problems.
- If you have some kind of kidney related issues, then it is best advised to discuss it with your nutritionist before starting a Keto diet. The high protein value will put a strain on the kidneys.

With that knowledge, you are pretty much set now to enter into the fantastical world of the Ketogenic diet!

Chapter 2: Start Your Day With These Keto Breakfast Meals

Keto Breakfast Tacos

If you are one of those people who used to love having taco nights or even "Taco Tuesdays" then you are going to absolutely fall in love with this recipe. This first recipe is dedicated to giving you more of an "Oomph" factor in your diet and give you something that you can feel hands on. Normally speaking, Ketogenic taco shells are made out of tortillas such as psyllium husks and flaxseed meal. While they do the job, they are never quite able to deliver the level of "crunch" of normal Tacos. Here, we are going to re-invent that by making our shells out of cheese!

Serving And Preparation Time

The following recipe is going to yield 3 servings and will take about 30-40 minutes to make and prepare.

Ingredients

- 1 cup of shredded mozzarella cheese
- 6 large eggs
- 2 tablespoons of butter
- 3 strips of bacon
- ½ of a small avocado
- 1 ounce of shredded cheddar cheese
- Salt as required
- Pepper as required

How to make

- For this recipe you are first going to need to cook up the bacon. Take out your oven tray and line it with a baking sheet using foil.
- Take the 3 strips of bacon and gently bake them in your oven at a temperature of 375F for 15-20 minutes.
- On the side, take a fresh pan and put it over medium heat. Toss in $1/3^{rd}$ of a cup of mozzarella.
- Wait for about 2-3 minutes until the edges of the cheese have obtained a nice brown texture.
- Take a spatula and slowly pull it up.
- Take the spatula and place it over a bowl so that it reaches from one side to the next. With tongs, pull up the cheese and drape it over the spatula so it hangs like a cloth on a clothesline.
- Keep repeating the process with the rest of the cheese.
- Take another pan and toss in the eggs and butter to cook them nicely, seasoning them with pepper and salt.
- Once the cheese has hardened, take them out and use a spoon to fill them up with the egg mixture.
- Take a few slices of avocado and add them in the shell as well.
- Make a final layer of the pieces of cooked bacon.
- Garnish by spreading cheddar cheese on top of the tacos.
- Serve it hot with cilantro and/or your favorite sauce.

Nutrition Values (3 Tacos)

- Calories: 443
- Fat: 36.2g
- Carbohydrate: 3g
- Protein: 25/7
- Dietary Fiber: 5g

Breakfast Keto Pizza Waffles

Sometimes people tend to get the strangest of cravings at the weirdest of times. Having a pizza for breakfast might sound really weird for the "normal" people out there, but those individuals who are on the Ketogenic diet are allowed sometimes to go for a well prepared healthy pizza such as the one here.

Serving And Preparation Time

The following recipe is going to yield 2 breakfast Keto pizza waffles and will take about 10-20 minutes to make and prepare.

Ingredients

- 4 large sized eggs
- 1 tablespoon of parmesan cheese
- 3 tablespoons of almond flour
- 1 tablespoon of psyllium husk powder
- 1 tablespoon of bacon grease
- 1 tablespoon of baking powder
- 1 teaspoon of Italian seasoning
- Salt as required
- Pepper as required
- ½ a cup of tomato sauce
- 3 ounces of cheddar cheese
- 14 slices of pepperoni

How to make

- Start this recipe by taking all the ingredients excluding the tomato sauce and cheese and tossing them into a container.
- Take an immersion blender and gently make sure to stir and blend everything until they are firmly

- mixed together. (Usually takes about 45 seconds max)
- Open up your waffle iron and add to it about half of the previously processed mixture.
- Let it cook for a while, keeping in mind that once it's ready, you will notice some steam coming off. Do the same until the batter is done.
- On top of the waffle, pour in about ¼ of a cup of sauce and toss in 1/5 ounce of cheese and some pepperoni.
- Put the processed waffle inside an oven and broil it for about 3-5 minutes.
- Once the cheese is molten, take it out and serve hot.

Nutrition Values (1 Pizza)

- Calories: 526
- Fat: 20
- Carbohydrate: 5g
- Protein: 29g
- Dietary Fiber: 11g

Keto Breakfast Burger

While this recipe might just a little bit heavy on calories, it still serves as a fine meal to set you up for the whole day if you are planning on missing out lunch or brunch.

Serving And Preparation Time

The following recipe is going to yield 2 Keto breakfast burgers and will take about 20-30 minutes to make and prepare.

Ingredients

- 4 ounces of sausage
- 2 ounces of pepper jack cheese
- 4 slices of bacon
- 2 large sized eggs
- 1 tablespoon of eggs
- 1 tablespoon of PB Fit powder
- Salt as required
- Pepper as required

How to make

- The first thing you are going to need to do for this recipe is prepare the bacon. Take out the cooking tray from your oven and lay the strips on top of a cookie sheet.
- Bake them for about 20-25 minutes at a temperature of 400F.
- Take a separate bowl and toss in the butter alongside the PB Fit powder. Keep them aside until they are re-hydrated.
- Take the sausages and mash them into patties. Then take a frying pan and cook them over medium-high heat making sure that both sides are brown.
- In the meantime, take some cheese and grate it.
- Once the patties are ready, toss in the cheese on top of them and cover them up.
- Gently remove the processed patties once the cheese has melted and fry an egg in the same pan, dropping the down the heat to a low level.
- Take a plate and combine everything on top of one another with a dash of rehydrated PB Fit as the cherry on top of everything.

Nutrition Values (Each Serving)

- Calories: 655
- Fat: 56g
- Carbohydrate: 3g
- Protein: 30.5g
- Dietary Fiber: 0.5g

Mini Pancake Donuts

National Donut day coming soon? Or just having a sudden craving for Donut in the morning? Take out your donut maker and batter up some of the most delicious yet easy to make Keto donuts ever!

Serving And Preparation Time

The following recipe is going to yield 22 donuts and will take about 25 minutes to make and prepare.

Ingredients

- 3 ounces of cream cheese
- 3 large sized eggs
- 4 tablespoons of almond flour
- 1 tablespoon of coconut flour
- 1 teaspoon of baking powder
- 1 teaspoon of vanilla extract
- 4 tablespoons of erythritol
- 10 drops of liquid stevia

How to make

- Take an immersion blender and toss in all of the ingredients in a bowl. Mix them up properly.
- You should blend them for about 45-60 seconds ensuring a nice and thick consistency.

- Now it's time to rack up your donut maker. Open it up and finely spray some coconut oil or non-stick oil to ensure that the donuts don't stick.
- Pour in the prepared batter and close the lid.
- It should take about 3 minutes for them to cook. Open the lid and flip them over. Cook them for another 2 minutes.
- Remove the donuts and keep repeating the process until done.
- Garnish them with your favorite topping and eat.

Nutrition Values (Each Donut)

- Calories: 32
- Fat: 2.7g
- Carbohydrate: 0.4g
- Protein: 1.4g
- Dietary Fiber: 0.4g

Cinnamon Roll Oatmeal

Oatmeal is are a long time favorite when it comes to a healthy breakfast for health buffs. But the problem with most oatmeal out there is that it is highly packed with carbs which is highly unsuitable for walkers of the Ketogenic path. The solution? Cinnamon oatmeal!

Serving And Preparation Time

The following recipe is going to yield 6 serving of cinnamon roll oatmeal and will take about 10-15 minutes to make and prepare.

Ingredients

- 1 cup of crushed pecans
- 1/3 cup of flax seed meal

- 1/3 cup of chia seeds
- ½ a cup of riced cauliflower
- 3 and a ½ cups of coconut milk
- 3 ounces of cream cheese
- 3 tablespoons of butter
- 1 and a ½ cups of cinnamon
- 3 tablespoons of maple flavor
- ½ a teaspoon of vanilla
- ¼ teaspoon of nutmeg
- ¼ teaspoon of allspice
- 3 tablespoons of powdered erythritol
- 10-15 drops of liquid stevia
- 1/8th teaspoon of xanthan gum

How to make

- For this recipe, start out by taking a bowl and tossing in the chia seeds alongside 1/3 cup of the ground flax seeds.
- Take a food processor and rice up about ½ a cup of cauliflower and set it aside.
- Take about a cup of raw pecans and put them in a Ziploc bag. Take a rolling pin to crush them nicely.
- Take a saucepan and put it over low heat. Toss in the crushed pecans.
- In another saucepan, pour in the coconut milk and warm it. Toss in the cauliflower and keep cooking it until it has reached its boiling point.
- Lower the heat and start adding the cinnamon, vanilla, maple flavor, allspice and nutmeg.
- Take a spice grinder and grind the Erythritol, powdering it.
- Toss in the powdered Erythritol to the milk mixture alongside some 10-15 drops of liquid stevia and keep stirring it.
- Toss in the chia and flaxseed and gently keep stirring it. Bear in mind that at this point, the whole mixture will thicken a lot.

- Once the whole mixture is hot again, toss in the previously processed pecans.
- Stir it and add in the cream, cream cheese and butter.
- Mix them all together and serve.
- The Xanthan gum is optional and you should add it only if you want your mixture to be a bit thicker.

Nutrition Values (Each Serving)

- Calories: 398
- Fat: 84g
- Carbohydrate: 3.1g
- Protein: 8.8g
- Dietary Fiber: 10.7g

Ham And Cheddar Chive Soufflé

Even Ketogenic followers sometimes desire to lean towards the more luxurious side of food. Start your day off with a nice little soufflé that is jam packed with fresh and savory flavors while keeping your calories at a minimum.

Serving And Preparation Time

The following recipe is going to yield 5 servings of ham cheddar chive soufflé and will take about 20-30 minutes to make and prepare.

Ingredients

- 3 tablespoons of olive oil
- ½ of a medium sized diced onion
- 1 and ½ teaspoons of minced garlic
- 6 ounces of cooked and cubed ham steak
- 1 tablespoon of butter

- 6 large sized eggs
- 1 cup of shredded cheddar cheese
- ½ a cup of double cream
- 2-3 tablespoons of freshly chopped chives
- ½ a teaspoon of Kosher salt
- ¼ a teaspoon of black pepper

How to make

- The first thing you are going to want to do is pre-heat your oven to a temperature of 400F.
- Prepare all the ingredients as mentioned in the ingredients list.
- Take a frying pan and pour in some olive oil, wait until hot.
- Toss in the onions and sauté them.
- Once the onions are softened, toss in the garlic and keep sautéing everything until the garlic has achieved a slightly brown texture.
- Take another bowl and toss in the eggs, double cream, chopped up chives and pepper.
- In this bowl, pour in the previously prepared garlic mixture and mix everything gently.
- Bake it in the pre-heated oven for about 20 minutes and serve hot.

Nutrition Values (Each Serving)

- Calories: 404
- Fat: 39.6g
- Carbohydrate: 3.5g
- Protein: 19.6g
- Dietary Fiber: 0.2g

Blackberry Pudding

If you are in the mode of taking a detour from meat based meals and want to go into the decadent world of sweets and berries, then go for this one! This blackberry pudding will refresh you in the morning and keep your carbs low at the same time.

Serving And Preparation Time

The following recipe is going to yield 2 serving of blackberry pudding and will take about 20-35 minutes to make and prepare.

Ingredients

- ¼ of a cup of coconut flour
- ¼ a teaspoon of baking powder
- 5 large egg yolks
- 2 tablespoons of coconut oil
- 2 tablespoons of butter
- 2 tablespoons of double cream
- 2 teaspoons of lemon juice
- Zest of 1 lemon
- 1/4 a cup of blackberries
- 2 tablespoons of Erythritol
- 10 drops of liquid stevia

How to make

- The first step here is to pre-heat your oven to a temperature of 350F,
- Take a bowl and separate the yolks from the egg whites.
- Put the coconut flour and baking powder in a separate bowl and set it aside as well.

- Take another small bowl and measure out the 2 tablespoons of coconut oil and 2 tablespoons of butter.
- Keep beating the egg yolks roughly followed by the addition of Erythritol and about 10 drops of liquid stevia. Keep beating them until fully combined.
- To that mixture, add the double cream, lemon juice and zest.
- Pour in the previous butter mixture and beat together until there are no lumps.
- Take the dry ingredients and sift them into the mixture and mix slowly until a nice batter forms.
- Take two ramekins and pour the batter into them.
- Using your finger, push some black berries on top of the batter.
- Place them inside your oven and bake them for around 20-25 minutes.
- Let them cool and you are done.

Nutrition Values (Each Pudding)

- Calories: 477.5
- Fat: 43.5g
- Carbohydrate: 5.5g
- Protein: 9g
- Dietary Fiber: 6.5g

Chapter 3: The Delightful Luncheon Recipes For Keto Lovers

Bacon Avocado And Chicken Sandwich

Taking a break from your heavy day, this bacon and chicken packed sandwich will help to provide you with enough energy to stay energetic until night while keeping your calorie count low.

Serving And Preparation Time

The following recipe is going to yield 2 serving of bacon and avocado sandwich and will take about 30-40 minutes to make and prepare.

Ingredients

For the Keto cloud bread

- 3 large sized eggs
- 3 ounces of cream cheese
- 1/8 teaspoon of cream cheese
- ¼ teaspoon of salt
- ½ teaspoon of garlic powder

For The Filling

- 1 tablespoon of mayonnaise
- 1 teaspoon of sriracha
- 2 slices of bacon
- 3 ounces of chicken
- 3 ounces of chicken
- 2 slices of pepper jack cheese
- 2 grape tomatoes

- ¼ medium avocado

How to make

- Begin by pre-heating your oven to a temperature of 300F.
- Take two bowls and break in 3 eggs and separate them.
- Into the bowl with the egg whites, pour in the tartar cream and use an electric mixer to whip up everything.
- In the other bowl with the egg yolks, toss in the cubed cream cheese and keep beating it until it is combined.
- Slowly fold the egg whites into the yolk mixture. Add half by half.
- Take a nice parchment paper lined baking sheet and scoop up about ¼ cup of the batter and place it on the sheet.
- Take a spatula and sprinkle in some garlic powder, and bake them for about 25 minutes.
- While it is baking, take a pan and toss in the chicken and bacon. Cook them with some pepper and salt.
- Once everything is ready, you are going to need to prepare your sandwich. Start off by combining the sriracha and mayonnaise.
- Spread them on the bottom part of the bread.
- Toss in the prepared chicken on top of the mayo mixture.
- Put in two slices of pepper jack cheese and cover it with the bacon.
- Add in some halved grape tomatoes and make a layer of mashed avocado as well.
- Season properly to taste and cover it up with the other bread.

Nutrition Values (Each Half)

- Calories: 361
- Fat: 28.3g
- Carbohydrate: 2g
- Protein: 22g
- Dietary Fiber: 2g

Cheese Stuffed Bacon Wrapped Hot Dogs

Who doesn't love cheese stuffed bacon wrapped hot dogs, right? These crisps are just the perfect blend of seasonings with a savory, rich, albeit a bit fatty flavor. If you are a cheese lover and you want to stay close to your Ketogenic roots, then look no further!

Serving And Preparation Time

The following recipe is going to yield 6 servings of cheese stuffed bacon wrapped hot dogs and will take about 35-45 minutes to make and prepare.

Ingredients

- 6 pieces of hot dog
- 12 slices of bacon
- 2 ounces of cheddar cheese
- ½ teaspoon of garlic powder
- ½ teaspoon of onion powder
- Salt as required
- Pepper as required

How to make

- Pre-heat your oven to a temperature of about 400F.
- Take the hot dog and make a slit into the sausage to make some space for the cheese.

- Slice about 2 ounces of cheddar cheese and stuff it inside the hot dog.
- Take the bacon and tightly wrap it around the hot dog.
- Once done, poke a toothpick from one end to the next to tightly secure the bacon in place.
- Set the prepared sausages on top of a cookie sheet and season them gently with onion, garlic powder and pepper and salt.
- Insert them in the pre-heated oven and bake them for about 35-40 minutes.
- Serve them to the audience with some creamed spinach and you are good to go!

Nutrition Values (Each Serving)

- Calories: 380
- Fat: 34.5g
- Carbohydrate: 0.3g
- Protein: 16.8g
- Dietary Fiber: 0.0g

Crispy Tofu and Bok Choy Salad

Combining the fine gooey and crunchy flavor of baked tofu with the super crunchy and distinctive bok choy marks a perfect balance in this salad in terms of being suitable for a Ketogenic diet and a mouth teaser.

Serving And Preparation Time

The following recipe is going to yield 3 servings of crispy tofu and bok choy salad and will take about 45-55 minutes to make and prepare.

Ingredients

For the oven baked tofu

- 15 ounce of extra firm tofu
- 1 tablespoon of soy sauce
- 1 tablespoon of sesame oil
- 1 tablespoon of water
- 2 teaspoons of minced garlic
- 1 tablespoon of rice wine vinegar
- Juice of ½ a lemon

For the bok choy salad

- 9 ounces of bok choy
- 1 stalk of green Onion
- 2 tablespoons of chopped cilantro
- 3 tablespoons of coconut oil
- 2 tablespoons of soy sauce
- 1 tablespoon of sambal oelek
- 1 tablespoon of peanut butter
- ½ lime
- 7 drops of liquid stevia

How to make

- Take the dry tofu and press it for about 6 hours.
- Take a bowl and toss in all of the ingredients required for the marinade which will include the sesame oil, soy sauce, water, garlic, lemon and vinegar.
- Take the pressed tofu and cut it up into square shapes then place it inside a plastic bag alongside the prepared marinade.
- Let it stay inside the fridge for at least 30 minutes, overnight at best.
- Pre-heat the oven to a temperature of 350F and place the tofu on a baking sheet. Bake for 30-35 minutes.

- Take another bowl and toss in the remaining ingredients for making the salad, excluding the bok choy.
- Toss in the cilantro and onion.
- Take the bok choy and slice it up into small pieces.
- Take the tofu out of the oven and assemble it with your salad.
- You are done!

Nutrition Values (Each Serving)

- Calories: 442
- Fat: 35g
- Carbohydrate: 5.7g
- Protein: 25g
- Dietary Fiber: 1.7g

Nasi Lemak

Originating from Indonesia, Singapore and Malaysia, this is an immensely popular rice dish that is as a matter of fact Malaysia's national dish. If you are in the mode to mimic one of Malaysia's most famous street dishes, then you are bound to give this a try.

Serving And Preparation Time

The following recipe is going to yield 2 servings of crispy tofu and bok choy salad and will take about 20 minutes to make and prepare.

Ingredients

For the sambal

- 1 large blended onion
- 0.35 ounces dried chilies
- 3 tablespoons of reduced sugar ketchup
- ½ a teaspoon of salt
- 2 tablespoons of coconut oil
- 1-2 drops of liquid sucralose

For the fried chicken

- 2 boneless chicken thighs
- ½ a teaspoon of curry powder
- ¼ a teaspoon of turmeric powder
- ½ a teaspoon of lime juice
- 1/8 a teaspoon of salt
- ½ a teaspoon of coconut oil

For The Nasi Lemak

- 3 tablespoons of coconut milk
- 3 slices of ginger
- ½ of a small shallot
- ¼ teaspoon salt
- 7 ounces of riced cauliflower
- 4 slices of cucumber

For The fried egg

- 1 large sized egg
- ½ tablespoon of unsalted butter

How to make

- Take the rice cauliflower and squeeze out the water thoroughly.
- Take the chicken thighs and marinade them with turmeric powder, curry powder, salt and lime juice.

- For the sambal you are going to need to chop up the onions and blend them until they are completely smooth.
- Take the dried chilis and remove the seeds.
- Let them boil for about 30 minutes until soft.
- Cool them down and blend them.
- Take a heated pan and melt down the coconut oil.
- Toss in the ingredients for the sambal adding just 1-2 drops of liquid sucralose.
- Once the chicken is marinated, fry it in a pan.
- Take another saucepan and boil the coconut milk alongside the shallots and ginger.
- Once the water has come to a bubbling heat, toss in the cauliflower and mix it up well.
- Serve it with 2 slices of cucumber alongside the fried egg and sambal/fried chicken.

Nutrition Values (Each Serving)

- Calories: 501
- Fat: 39.9g
- Carbohydrate: 6.9g
- Protein: 28.1g
- Dietary Fiber: 2.8g

Jalapeno Popper Mug Cake

If you are looking for something different to try out, then you can go with this nice mug cake which will help you to fill up your empty stomach within just a few minutes. This is somewhat a cross between a sandwich and a cake which in reality tastes as delicious as you might think.

Serving And Preparation Time

The following recipe is going to yield 1 serving of jalapeno popper mug cake and will take about 10-15 minutes to make and prepare.

Ingredients

- 2 tablespoons of almond flour
- 1 tablespoon of golden flaxseed meal
- 1 tablespoon of cutter
- 1 tablespoon of cream cheese
- 1 large size egg
- 1 piece of sliced and cooked bacon
- ½ of a jalapeno pepper
- ½ teaspoon of baking powder
- ¼ teaspoon of salt

How to make

- Take a frying pan and place it over medium heat.
- Take the sliced bacon and cook it until it has a crispy texture.
- Take a container and mix all of the ingredients together.
- Clean the sides.
- Microwave the whole dish for 75 seconds putting it on power 10.
- Gently tap the cup against a plate to take out the mug cake.
- Garnish it with some jalapenos and serve.

Nutrition Values (1 Mug)

- Calories: 429
- Fat: 38g
- Carbohydrate: 4.2g
- Protein: 16.5g
- Dietary Fiber: 4.2g

Chicken Enchilada Soup

Amidst a number of solid savories, here we have a nice and heart melting soup that is packed with hints of spice and creaminess. The chunks of chicken will give you an added flavor. But the best part of this dish is the fact it is able to beautifully encompass the flavors of an enchilada without the tortilla and extra carb value.

Serving And Preparation Time

The following recipe is going to yield 4 servings of chicken enchilada soup and will take about 40-50 minutes to make and prepare.

Ingredients

- 3 tablespoons of olive oil
- 3 stalks of diced celery
- 1 medium sized diced red bell pepper
- 2 teaspoons of minced garlic
- 4 cups of chicken broth
- 1 cup of diced tomatoes
- 8 ounces of cream cheese
- 6 ounces of shredded chicken
- 2 teaspoons of cumin
- 1 teaspoon of oregano
- 1 teaspoon of chili powder
- ½ teaspoon of cayenne pepper
- ½ a cup of chopped cilantro
- ½ of a juiced medium lime

How to make

- The first step here is to take a frying pan and heat some oil.

- Toss in the pepper and celery and cook until the celery is softened.
- Toss in the tomatoes and let them cook for about 3 minutes more.
- Into the pan, add in the spices and mix them together.
- Pour in the cilantro and chicken broth and slowly bring the mixture to a boil.
- Once the water starts bubbling, you are going to need to lower the temperature and let it simmer for about 20 minutes
- After 20 minutes you are going to toss in the cream cheese and bring it to a boil again. This time you are going to reduce the heat and simmer it for another 25 minutes.
- Take the chicken, shred it and toss it into the pot.
- Squeeze in just ½ of a lime over to the top.
- Stir everything and finally, top it off with some sprinkles of shredded cheese, sour cream or cilantro.

Nutrition Values (Each Serving)

- Calories: 345
- Fat: 31.3g
- Carbohydrate: 6g
- Protein: 13.3g
- Dietary Fiber: 1.8g

Thai Peanut Shrimp Curry

This is a very interesting amalgam of multiple flavors coming from the added peanut butter, coconut, cilantro and lime. When you take your first spoonful, you are bound to get a hint of coconut and lime which will evolve into a more powerful and delicious combination.

Serving And Preparation Time

The following recipe is going to yield 2 servings of Thai peanut shrimp curry soup and will take about 10-20 minutes to make and prepare.

Ingredients

- 2 tablespoons of green curry paste
- 1 cup of vegetable stock
- 1 cup of coconut milk
- 6 ounces of pre-cooked shrimp
- 5 ounces of broccoli florets
- 3 tablespoons of chopped cilantro
- 2 tablespoons of coconut oil
- 1 tablespoon of peanut butter
- 1 tablespoon of soy sauce
- Juice of ½ a lime
- 1 medium sized spring onion chopped up
- 1 teaspoon of crushed roasted garlic
- 1 teaspoon of minced garlic
- 1 teaspoon of fish sauce
- ½ teaspoon of turmeric
- ¼ teaspoon of xanthan gum
- ½ a cup of sour cream

How to make

- Start by putting a pan over medium heat and add 2 tablespoons of coconut oil.
- Once the oil is melted, toss in the minced ginger and chopped up spring onion. Let them cook for about a minute before putting in the turmeric and curry paste.
- Add about 1 tablespoon of soy sauce, peanut butter and fish sauce and mix them well.

- Then add in a cup of vegetable stock and just a cup of coconut milk.
- Stir them well before adding the green curry paste.
- Simmer them for a while.
- Add in about ¼ teaspoon of xanthan gum to the curry and mix it properly/
- After a while you will notice that the curry will begin to thicken, that will be the moment when you will need to throw in the florets and stir them finely.
- Add in the fresh chopped cilantro.
- Once the consistency is fine, you are going to need to toss in the weighed pre-cooked shrimps and add the lime juice.
- Let the mixture simmer for a few minutes and season it with pepper and salt as required.
- Finally, serve it hot alongside just a ¼ a cup of sour cream with each serving.

Nutrition Values (Each Serving)

- Calories: 455
- Fat: 31.5g
- Carbohydrate: 8.9g
- Protein: 27g
- Dietary Fiber: 4.8g

Chapter 4: Meals For When You Are About To Sleep, Your Dinner

Keto Sushi

Sushi is definitely an instant classic when it comes to food lovers. Usually these are made primarily out of some kind of meat, but this time they are made using a unique blend of broccoli, making it suitable for any Ketogenic lover.

Serving And Preparation Time

The following recipe is going to yield 3 servings of Ketogenic sushi and will take about 10-20 minutes to make and prepare.

Ingredients

- 16 ounces of cauliflower
- 6 ounces of softened cream cheese
- 1-2 tablespoons of rice vinegar
- 1 tablespoon of soy sauce
- 5 sheets of Nori
- 1 6 inch piece of cucumber
- ½ of a medium avocado
- 5 ounces of smoked salmon

How to make

- The first step here is to put the cauliflower into a processor and blend it into rice sized pieces.
- Take the cucumber and slice it at each end. Then place the cucumber upright and slice off the sides.

- Throw away the middle portion then take the strips and place them in a fridge.
- Place a pan on top of a high flame, toss in the cauliflower rice and cook it.
- Season it with some soy sauce.
- When the rice is done, take it out and dry it.
- Take a bowl and toss in the cream cheese along with the rice vinegar.
- Mix them properly and set it in a fridge.
- In the meantime, the rice mixture will cool down, now you are going to need to add strips of avocado.
- Finally, put the nori sheets down on a bamboo roller and cover them up with saran wrap.
- Gently spread the cauliflower rice mixture and roll up the nori sheet after adding the other fillings.
- Serve well.

Nutrition Values (Each 1 and a half roll)

- Calories: 353
- Fat: 25.7g
- Carbohydrate: 5.7g
- Protein: 28.3g
- Dietary Fiber: 8g

Walnut Crusted Salmon

When you are on a Ketogenic diet with strong devotion, you are definitely in it because you want to stay healthy. It has been proven that fatty fish helps to decrease cholesterol levels and improve overall health. These benefits make this a very easy and cheap recipe which can be made within a very short time.

Serving And Preparation Time

The following recipe is going to yield 2 servings of walnut crusted salmon and will take about 15-20 minutes to make and prepare.

Ingredients

- ½ a cup of walnuts
- 2 tablespoons of sugar free maple syrup
- ½ a tablespoon of Dijon mustard
- ¼ sprig of dill
- 2 pieces of 3 ounce salmon fillets
- 1 tablespoon of olive oil
- Salt as needed
- Pepper as needed

How to make

- The first step here it to pre-heat your oven to a temperature of 350F.
- Add in just half a cup of walnuts to your food processor.
- To the walnuts, pour in the maple syrup and spices.
- Then pour in the mustard.
- Blend the whole mixture in the food processor until a consistency similar to paste has been achieved.
- Take a pan and heat it up with just a tablespoon of oil.
- When it is very hot, toss in the salmon fillets and let them sear for about 3 minutes.
- Toss in the walnuts on the upper side of the fillet.
- Once seared, take the fillets to the pre-heated oven and bake them for about 8 minutes. Serve them with a fresh bunch of spinach, and if you prefer then you can also go for a few sprinkles of paprika.

Nutrition Values (Each serving)

- Calories: 373
- Fat: 43g
- Carbohydrate: 3g
- Protein: 20g
- Dietary Fiber: 1g

Slow Cooker Braised Oxtail

If you are not already aware of it, then you should know that oxtail is a very juicy and tender dish! The only drawback is that it takes a long time to cook. That is exactly why for this recipe we are going to be using a slow cooker. With an increasing popularity this is a must try dish for Keto lovers.

Serving And Preparation Time

The following recipe is going to yield 3 servings of Keto slow cooker braised oxtail and will take about 6-7 hours to make and prepare.

Ingredients

- 2 pounds of oxtails with bones in
- 2 cups of beef broth
- 1/3 cup of butter
- 2 tablespoons of soy sauce
- 1 tablespoon of fish sauce
- 3 tablespoons of tomato paste
- 1 teaspoon of onion powder
- 1 teaspoon of minced garlic
- ½ teaspoon of ground ginger
- 1 teaspoon of dried thyme
- Salt as required

- Pepper as required
- ½ a teaspoon of guar gum

How to make

- The first step here is to heat up the beef broth on a stove and combine it with the fish sauce, soy sauce, butter and tomato paste.
- Once done, gently transfer it to the slow cooker and mix everything including the oxtails.
- Carefully season the oxtails and broth with minced garlic, onion powder, dried thyme and ground ginger.
- Add pepper and salt as needed.
- Cook it on low for about 6-7 hours.
- Drain the oxtail once the cooking is done and serve dry if preferred.
- If you want the gravy to be a little bit thicker, then you can go for an immersion blender. Just place the leftover juices from the cooker and use some guar gum while blending the mixture.

Nutrition Values (Each serving)

- Calories: 433
- Fat: 29.7g
- Carbohydrate: 3.2g
- Protein: 28.3g
- Dietary Fiber: 1g

Nacho Chicken Casserole

A South Western variation of shepherd's pie is not something to take lightly. This is a dish that is crammed with gooey cheesy delight. But the fact the whole dish is created in the form of a casserole makes it perfectly suitable for being a Keto recipe with a fine balance of sweetness and acidity.

Serving And Preparation Time

The following recipe is going to yield 6 serving of nacho chicken casserole and will take about 20-30 minutes to make and prepare.

Ingredients

- 1.75 pounds of boneless and skinless chicken thighs
- 1 and a ½ teaspoons of chili seasoning
- 2 tablespoons of olive oil
- 4 ounces of cream cheese
- 4 ounces of cheddar cheese
- 1 cup of green chilies and tomatoes
- ¼ cup of sour cream
- 16 ounces of frozen cauliflower
- 1 medium sized jalapeno pepper
- Salt as required
- Pepper as required

How to make

- The first step here is to pre-heat your oven to a temperature of 375F.
- After that, take kitchen shears and chop up your chicken into chunk sized pieces.
- Season the chunked chicken with pepper, salt and chili seasoning.
- Take a pan over medium-high heat and toss in the chicken thighs, cook them until they have gained a nice brown texture.
- In that pan, toss in the sour cream, cream cheese and about ¾ of the cheddar cheese.

- Stir everything gently until the butter has completely melted.
- To the mixture, add in some green chilis and combine them together.
- Take a casserole dish and add in the prepared chicken mixture.
- On the side, microwave the frozen cauliflower to cook it properly.
- Take an immersion blender and combine everything with the cheese to give it a nice mashed potato consistency.
- Season the mixture with some pepper and salt.
- Take the jalapenos and cut them into small chunks.
- Sprinkle them on top of the casserole.
- Bake for about 20 minutes.
- You could also throw in some fresh Cilantro.

Nutrition Values (Each serving)

- Calories: 426
- Fat: 32.2g
- Carbohydrate: 4.3g
- Protein: 30.8g
- Dietary Fiber: 1.7g

Ketogenic Grilled Short Ribs

Korean style BBQ is a very famous dish all around the world. Just because you are a Keto follower doesn't mean that you are going to have to let go of this as well! Just follow the recipe and you will be able to craft yourself a nice inexpensive, delicious and tender meat dish!

Serving And Preparation Time

The following recipe is going to yield 4 servings of Asian grilled Keto short ribs and will take about 60-70 minutes to make and prepare.

Ingredients

For the ribs and marinade

- 6 large pieces of short ribs
- ¼ cup of soy sauce
- 2 tablespoons of rice vinegar
- 2 tablespoons of fish sauce

For the spice rub

- 1 teaspoon of ground ginger
- ½ teaspoon of onion powder
- ½ teaspoon of minced garlic
- ½ teaspoon of red pepper flakes
- ½ a teaspoon of sesame seeds
- ¼ teaspoon of cardamom
- 1 tablespoon of salt

How to make

- Firstly you are going to want to take a pot and pour in the rice vinegar, soy sauce and fish sauce.
- Take a casserole dish and set the ribs in it until the edges have been raised.
- Pour in the marinade and let the ribs sit for about 45-60 minutes.
- Combine all the ingredients of the spice rub.
- Empty the marinade from the casserole and pour in the marinade to the spicy mixture on either side of the ribs.

- Fire up your grill and grill the ribs for about 3-5 minutes.
- Finally serve it up with your favorite side dish of vegetables.

Nutrition Values (Each serving)

- Calories: 417
- Fat: 31.8g
- Carbohydrate: 0.9g
- Protein: 29.5g
- Dietary Fiber: 0g

Oven Baked Turkey Leg

Thanksgiving is not the only period of time when you are allowed to go for turkey! Sometimes you might just feel like eating a turkey fry after coming home from work or school! This recipe is a Ren Fest inspired meal which is just perfect for friendly get-togethers and gatherings.

Serving And Preparation Time

The following recipe is going to yield 4 servings of oven roasted turkey legs and will take about 70 minutes to make and prepare.

Ingredients

- 2 medium sized turkey legs
- 2 tablespoons of duck fat
- 2 teaspoons of salt
- ½ a teaspoon of pepper
- ¼ teaspoon of cayenne pepper
- ½ a teaspoon of onion powder

- ½ a teaspoon of dried thyme
- ½ teaspoon of Ancho chili powder
- 1 teaspoon of Liquid Smoke
- 1 teaspoon of Worcestershire sauce

How to make

- For this recipe all you are going to have to do is first take a simple bowl and pour in the wet ingredients to mix them up.
- Take the turkey legs and pat them using a dry towel.
- Gently rub the turkey legs with proper seasoning.
- Pre-heat your oven to a temperature of 350F.
- Take a cast iron skillet or a frying pan and drop in 2 tablespoons of fat.
- The temperature should be around medium-high. The oil will soon start to smoke.
- At this point, you are going to add the turkey legs to the pan and let them sear for about 1 to 2 minutes. Let them sear on both sides.
- Gently place them inside the oven, at a temperature of 350F for around 50-60 minutes.
- Once done, remove them and serve them hot!

Nutrition Values (Each serving)

- Calories: 382
- Fat: 22.5g
- Carbohydrate: 0.8g
- Protein: 44g
- Dietary Fiber: 0g

Italian Stuffed Meatballs

Although it's nothing much fancy, this simple meatball recipe is highly delicious and easy to make in the sense that it takes only 30 minutes to make, using only ingredients that are available in any household kitchen. Since you are looking for something easy, this is your one stop shop.

Serving And Preparation Time

The following recipe is going to yield 4 servings of stuffed meatballs and will take about 30 minutes to make and prepare.

Ingredients

- 1 and a ½ pounds of ground beef
- 1 teaspoon of oregano
- ½ teaspoon of Italian seasoning
- 2 teaspoons of minced garlic
- ½ teaspoon of onion powder
- 3 tablespoons of tomato paste
- 3 tablespoons of Flaxseed Meal
- 2 large eggs
- ½ a cup of sliced olives
- ½ a cup of mozzarella cheese
- 1 teaspoon of Worcestershire sauce
- Salt as required
- Pepper as required

How to make

- The first step here is to take a large bowl and toss in the ground beef, Italian seasoning, oregano, onion powder and garlic.
- Use your hands to properly mix them altogether.

- To that mixture, add the tomato paste, eggs, Worcestershire sauce and flaxseed. Mix them together again.
- Once done, take the pieces of olives and sliced them up. Toss the sliced olives with shredded slices of mozzarella cheese.
- Take the mixture and roll it up into balls.
- Pre-heat the oven to a temperature of 400F.
- Place the balls on top of foil and bake them for about 20 minutes.
- Take them out and serve!

Nutrition Values (Each serving)

- Calories: 382
- Fat: 22.5g
- Carbohydrate: 0.8g
- Protein: 44g
- Dietary Fiber: 0g

Chapter 5: A Few Desserts For The Sweet Tooth Out There

Mini Vanilla Cloud Cupcakes

Love cupcakes? Love guilt-free cupcakes? Then you are in for a treat! These delicately crafted low carb vanilla muffins are to die for when you are looking to end a nice meal with something soft and mouthwatering.

Serving And Preparation Time

The following recipe is going to yield 8 serving of vanilla cloud cupcakes and will take about 30-40 minutes to make and prepare.

Ingredients

For the cake

- 6 large sized separated eggs
- 6 tablespoons of cream cheese at room temperature
- ½ teaspoon of tartar cream
- 2 teaspoons of vanilla extract
- ¼ cup of granulated stevia/erythritol mixture

For the frosting

- 16 ounces of softened cream cheese
- 2 tablespoons of softened butter
- 1/3 cup of granulated stevia/erythritol mix
- 1 tablespoon of vanilla extract

How to make

- Start this recipe off by pre-heating your oven to a temperature of 300F.
- Take 2 muffin tins and spray them with non-stick spray.
- Take a bowl and toss in the cream cheese, sweetener, egg yolks and vanilla extract.
- Keep beating them together until they have acquired a nice and smooth consistency.
- Take a separate bowl and gently whip the cream of tartar and egg whites using an electric mixer.
- Gently take the whipped mixture and pour it into the yolk mixture.
- Scoop up the mixture and place it in the muffin tins.
- Place the tin inside the oven and let them cook for about 30-35 minutes.
- When done, remove the cakes from the muffin tin and place them on a rack to cool.
- Take a medium sized bowl and combine all of the ingredients listed under the "frosting" section.
- Keep beating the mixture using an electric mixer until a smooth consistency has been achieved.
- Fill up the whipped cream in a bag and pipe some mixture onto a muffin, place a muffin on top and add more whip, creating three layers.
- Serve and eat!

Nutrition Values (Each Cake)

- Calories: 347
- Fat: 30g
- Carbohydrate: 3.4g
- Protein: 9g
- Dietary Fiber: 3.5g

Bake Free Coconut Cashew Bars

Keto friendly bars are extremely rare in this world where protein and low carb bars are found everywhere. This recipe is designed to save you from that trouble and get the benefit of a nutrition bar that will give you the required dose of nutrients alongside the flavor of a dessert.

Serving And Preparation Time

The following recipe is going to yield 8 serving of bake free coconut cashew bars and will take about 10-15 minutes to make and prepare.

Ingredients

- 1 cup of almond flour
- ¼ cup of melted butter
- ¼ cup of sugar free maple syrup
- 1 teaspoon of cinnamon
- 1 pinch of salt
- ½ a cup of cashew nuts
- ¼ cup of shredded coconut

How to make

- For this recipe firstly you are going to need to combine the melted butter and almond flour by tossing them into a large bowl.
- To that mix, toss in the cinnamon, sugar free maple syrup and salt. Mix them up well.
- Once done, add the coconut which you have shredded previously and mix it again.

- Take the cashew nuts and roughly chop about ½ cup of them. Throw them into the prepared dough and mix everything properly.
- Line a baking dish using a parchment paper and spread out the dough in even layers.
- If you want you can garnish it with some cinnamon and shredded coconut for added taste and beauty.
- Place the whole dish in a fridge and cool it for about 2 hours, then slice them up into nice bars when ready.

Nutrition Values (Each Serving)

- Calories: 189
- Fat: 17.6g
- Carbohydrate: 4g
- Protein: 4g
- Dietary Fiber: 2.1g

Choco Peanut Tarts

Just because you are following a Ketogenic diet plan doesn't mean that you have to relinquish chocolate and peanut butter from your life! This recipe is a prime example that even Keto followers can easily have a guilt free dessert packed with the delight of chocolate and peanut butter while being low in calories.

Serving And Preparation Time

The following recipe is going to yield 4 serving of chocolate and peanut butter tarts and will take about 30-40 minutes to make and prepare.

Ingredients

For the crust

- ¼ cup of flaxseed
- 2 tablespoons of almond flour
- 1 tablespoon of erythritol
- 1 large egg white

For the top layer

- 1 medium sized avocado
- 4 tablespoons of cocoa powder
- ¼ cup of erythritol
- ½ teaspoon of vanilla extract
- ½ teaspoon of cinnamon
- 2 tablespoons of double cream

Middle layer

- 4 tablespoons of peanut butter
- 2 tablespoons of butter

How to make

- Preheat the oven to a temperature of 350F.
- Take a separate bowl and toss in the flaxseed and grind them until they are firmly ground.
- To the flaxseed mix, add the rest of the ingredients listed under the crust.
- Take a tart pan and pour in the crust mixture, then put it inside the oven and bake it for 8 minutes.
- Take another bowl and prepare the top layer by combining all of the ingredients listed under the crust. Blend them to get a creamy and smooth mixture.
- Once the crust inside the oven is complete, take it out and let it cool.

- For the peanut butter layer, you are going to need to take another bowl and melt the peanut butter and butter mixture in your microwave.
- Gently pour in the molten peanut butter mixture on top of your crust layer and leave it for 30 minutes to settle down.
- Over the peanut butter layer, pour in the chocolate avocado layer and let the whole tart refrigerate for an hour.
- Take it out from the fridge and serve.

Nutrition Values (Each Half Tart)

- Calories: 305
- Fat: 26.8g
- Carbohydrate: 3.9g
- Protein: 9.8g
- Dietary Fiber: 6.6g

Pumpkin Pecan Pie Ice Cream

Just thinking about this recipe will water the mouth of any individual. A combination of two thanksgiving dishes, namely a pecan pie and pumpkin pie! This ice cream is an exquisite and delightful mixture that is bursting with savory flavor. A perfect showstopper for a Ketogenic follower.

Serving And Preparation Time

The following recipe is going to yield 4 servings of pumpkin pecan pie Keto ice cream and will take about 10-15 minutes to make and prepare.

Ingredients

- ½ a cup of cottage cheese
- ½ a cup of pumpkin puree
- 1 teaspoon of pumpkin spice
- 2 cups of coconut milk
- ½ a teaspoon of xanthan gum
- 3 large sized egg yolks
- 1/3 cup of erythritol
- 20 drops of liquid stevia
- 1 teaspoon of maple extract
- ½ a cup of toasted and chopped up pecans
- 2 tablespoons of salted butter

How to make

- The first step of this recipe is to take a pan and put it on the stove. Toss in the toasted pecans and butter and leave the pan over a low heat for the butter to melt.
- Take a container and toss in the rest of the listed ingredients and blend them properly using an immersion blender.
- Add the mixture to an ice cream machine.
- Toss the butter and pecan mixture into the ice cream machine.
- Churn everything properly following the instructions of your ice cream machine and serve

Nutrition Values (Each Cup)

- Calories: 248
- Fat: 22.3g
- Carbohydrate: 4.3g
- Protein: 6.5g
- Dietary Fiber: 2.9g

Conclusion

I would like to take a moment here and end the book on a thank you note.

I really do hope that you enjoyed reading this and had a nice time exploring through all of the different recipes. From this point on, I encourage you to explore the world of the Ketogenic diet even further as you have just reached the tip of the iceberg here!

May you stay safe and healthy!

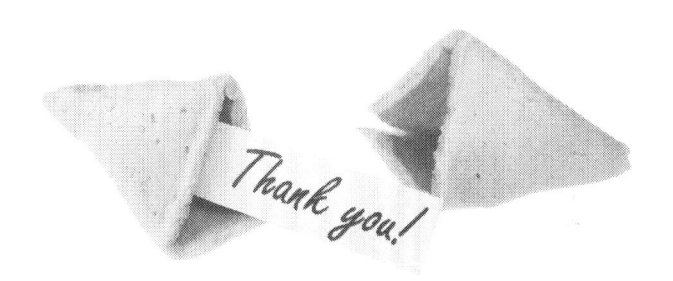

Made in the USA
San Bernardino, CA
07 February 2017